the fast
800
Health
journal

the fast
800
Health journal

DR CLARE BAILEY
Foreword by DR MICHAEL MOSLEY

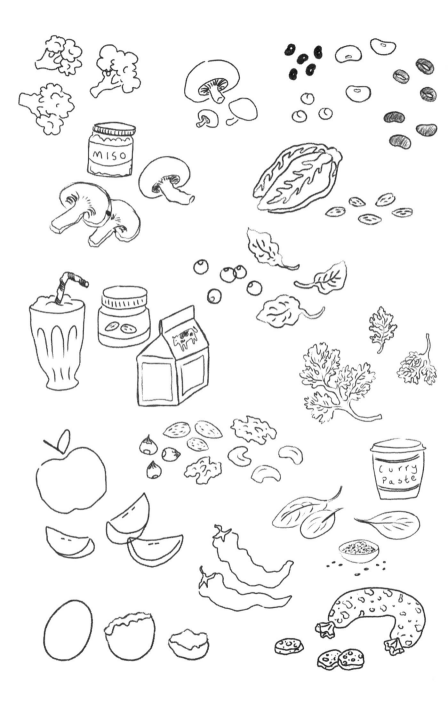

MISO

Curry
Paste

This book belongs to

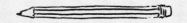

Foreword

I have been hugely enthusiastic about the benefits of intermittent fasting ever since 2012, when I lost a lot of weight, fast, and managed to reverse my type 2 diabetes on a regime I called the 5:2 diet. A great deal of new science has emerged since then, and in my most recent book, *The Fast 800*, I have pulled together the best of this research into a new programme, which still incorporates the 5:2 but is based on, among other things, more manageable 800-calorie fast days.

As we all know, losing weight is not just about 'calories in and calories out'. We all have different needs and different demands in our lives. In the end, the best diet is the one you can stick to and which fits best in your life.

This is where food journaling comes in. Food is embedded in almost every aspect of our lives – not just as fuel to keep us going, but as a way of bringing people together, a way of showing love and receiving it. On the flip side, food can become a false friend – something we turn to as a source of comfort when we feel down or stressed, and which we can easily become unhappily addicted to and dependent upon. We are surrounded by constant temptation, which is hard to resist. On top of this, the actual foods we eat (processed and heavily promoted by the food industry) can hijack our brains and our hormones.

Keeping a food journal has been shown to be a particularly useful tool for personal change – not only to help with weight loss, but to make us generally more mindful of what we eat, how we eat it, and why.

A study by Kaiser Permanente's Center for Health Research, one of the largest and longest weight-loss maintenance trials ever conducted, found that those who kept daily food records lost twice as much weight as those who didn't. It seems that the simple act of writing down what you eat (and, don't forget, drink) heightens awareness and encourages people to consume fewer calories.

At the same time, keeping a daily diary can encourage better habits. Very often we forget about the little snacks and extras that we graze on in down time. But just the knowledge that you are writing down your daily consumption means that you are less likely to pick up a bag of crisps to keep you going before supper, or a bar of chocolate at the till when you do your weekly shop.

Keeping track of your location when you eat something, the time of day, and your mood helps you identify the triggers to unhealthy eating and can reveal how stress, work, or certain people affect your food choices. For example, if you reach for a biscuit each time you enter the office, then you may deduce that stressful environments cause you to crave sugary foods. If you eat every meal standing up, then you're probably rushing and eating more calories than if you sat down and took your time.

The important thing is that the diary is an honest and accurate record. A few years ago I made a film with an overweight woman who couldn't understand why she wasn't losing weight. We asked her to keep a food diary for a couple of weeks. At the same time we gave her a drink containing something called "doubly labelled water", which contains an element that allows you to trace how many calories you are using up, and therefore how many you are *really* consuming. When we totted up her diary it came to less than 1500 calories. The doubly labelled water technique suggested she was consuming almost twice that.

Before you tut-tut, it's easily done. As someone who craves chocolate and has been found (rarely!) gouging cheesecake straight out of the freezer late at night, I am well aware of how strong temptation can be.

We have organised this food diary to give you as many helpful prompts as possible. I do hope you enjoy using it and find it helpful on your weight loss journey. The more mindful we are of our daily lives, the happier and healthier we are.

WHAT IS THE FAST 800?

The Fast 800 has three stages:

The Very Fast 800 – rapid weight loss
The New 5:2 – intermittent fasting
The Way of Life – maintenance

What all these stages have in common is that they are based on 800-calorie fast days. That's because 800 is the magic number when it comes to successful dieting – it's high enough to be manageable and sustainable but low enough to trigger a range of desirable metabolic changes.

The choice you have to make is how intensively you want to do the programme – i.e. how many 800-calorie days to include each week from the start, and how to adjust these as you progress.

For rapid weight loss, as long as it is safe for you to do it (see page 13), 800 calories a day, every day, is what you should be aiming at. This is a regimen that has been shown to be safely sustainable for weeks and even up to three months. You might want to take this approach if you have a lot of weight to lose; if you have pre-diabetes or type 2 diabetes; if you are in a hurry or perhaps because you have hit a weight loss plateau.

However, not everyone can or will want to stick to 800 calories a day for long. You might just want to use it to kick-start things, and after a few weeks move on to the

"New 5:2". Will you still lose weight, fast? Yes, particularly if you start with the rapid weight loss approach, and then move on to fasting just two days a week.

Once you have hit your goals, you can graduate to Stage 3, where you stick to a lowish carb Mediterranean-style diet as a Way of Life. You no longer need to count calories at this stage, but do be careful about your portion size – if you return to your old ways you will return to your pre-diet body. The key is to keep on top of things: weigh yourself weekly; don't worry if you have had a busy social time and you have put on a few pounds, but act quickly to shed them – add in a fast 800 day, or go back on to the New 5:2 for a week or two.

What to eat

The Fast 800 is based on a low-carb, moderately high-protein Mediterranean-style diet. One rich in healthy natural fats, nuts and fish, as well as veggies and legumes, which are packed with disease-fighting vitamins and minerals.

The reason I am so keen on this way of eating is not just because it tastes great but because there is so much solid evidence that adopting this lifestyle will cut your risk of cancer, heart disease, type 2 diabetes, depression and dementia. It will also help you maintain your muscle mass and stop your metabolic rate from crashing as you lose weight. This means you will find it much easier to keep the weight off, long term.

Please be aware that the Mediterranean diet I'm writing about is the traditional one of the people who lived around the Mediterranean Sea before they, like so much of the planet, adopted junk food. It is not the sort of food that you would typically associate with your holidays in Italy or Greece. It does not, for instance, include lots of pizza and pasta, or the sort of sticky puddings you might be offered in a Greek restaurant.

When to eat

One of the new elements I introduced with the Fast 800 programme is a popular idea called Time Restricted Eating, or TRE, and we have included a space in your daily journal to record your progress with this.

TRE involves eating all your calories within a relatively narrow time window each day, usually 8 to 12 hours. This extends the length of your normal overnight fast (the time when you are asleep and not eating) and gives your body an opportunity to burn fat and do essential repairs.

You can start doing TRE by simply having your evening meal a bit earlier and your breakfast a bit later. That way you extend your normal overnight fast by a few hours. Once you have got used to this you can move to the 14:10 (where you eat all your calories in a 10-hour window, such as between 10am and 8pm, and fast for 14 hours) or even, like Hugh Jackman, to the 16:8. We have included a place for you to record your daily TRE in the journal. Just note whether you have done a 10-, 12- or 14-hour fasting window on the circles provided.

OTHER PILLARS OF
THE FAST 800 PROGRAMME

Getting active

We all know how important it is to do exercise and remain active, but knowing something and doing it are very different things. I don't particularly like exercise, and I hate the gym, so I have found ways to make myself do what I need to do to keep myself healthy and happy, to sleep better and keep my brain in decent shape.

We have included a specific box in this diary so you can record your daily activity (whether this is going for a short jog, walking around the block, doing the cleaning or repeatedly getting up from your chair). Many of us like to think that we do quite a lot of exercise, but seeing it written down in black and white can be an eye opener: was it really three weeks ago that I last went to the gym?

Noting what works and what doesn't

The point here is to be mindful of your routine and how you are coping. So if something has gone well on a particular day, note it down. It doesn't have to be anything major: maybe after going for a pre-breakfast run in the sun you felt particularly energised, or you discovered a great, easy recipe that you found satisfying or you were simply able to distract yourself by keeping very busy. This focuses your attention on the positive and is a good way to lift your mood and bolster confidence. We have provided a space for this as part of your daily diary routine.

Be clear about your GOALs

Get: What do you want to get out of this diet? Weight loss? Better blood sugars? A smaller waist? To come off medication?

Opportunities: What resources and opportunities are available to help you succeed? Friends and family? Professionals? Diet buddy? An online forum like the one at www.thefast800.com?

Approach: How do you intend to approach this diet? What steps do you need to take to help you succeed? What has worked in the past? What will help keep you on track? Which combination of 800-calorie days could work for you?

Look for successes: Take one day at a time – look for small changes in your measurements, how you feel, your energy levels, your activity levels. Notice and celebrate small positive changes.

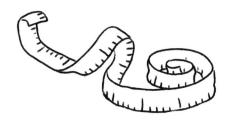

What about meal replacement shakes?
Some people find using meal replacement shakes can
really help on fast days, particularly at the start, because
then you don't have to think about what to buy and cook
for every meal. It also means you don't have to worry about
counting calories or getting in all your essential nutrients
for those meals. Plus, they can be a quick and easy solution
when dashing out first thing in the morning or to take to
work for lunch.

We are very pragmatic on this. If you do want to go
the shake route, you should aim for something low in
carbs, and containing plenty of protein, enough fat and
decent amounts of fibre (see www.thefast800.com for
suggested brands which do not have too much added sugar
and are suited to a low-carb Mediterranean way of eating).
However, if you would like to whizz up your own, we have
some tasty recipes on our website. Do try them out.

Remember to record your shake and calorie count in
the breakfast, lunch or dinner slots in your journal in the
normal way.

Cautions & exclusions
This diet is not suitable for under-18s, or if you're
breastfeeding, pregnant or undergoing fertility treatment.
Do not do it if you are underweight or have an eating
disorder. Discuss with your GP if you are on medication
or if you have a medical condition, including diabetes,
low or high blood pressure, retinopathy or epilepsy.
Nor should you do this is you are frail, unwell or
whilst doing endurance exercise. (For more detailed
information see https://thefast800.com/faqs/)

Before you start

It's great that you are planning to make constructive changes to your diet and lifestyle with the Fast 800. Before embracing a significant change, it helps to be clear in your mind as to why you are doing it and what you want to achieve.

Think about what difference doing this diet will make to you. Why does doing this matter to you? It may be because you want to get into that outfit for your daughter's wedding, or to lose the spare tyre, feel fitter, be able to chase your grandchildren in the park or to reduce your blood sugars and reverse your diabetes. We will ask you to write this down.

And when it comes to what targets you want to achieve, this should include a limited number of measurable improvements such as getting down to a specific target weight, reducing your waist measurement or improving your blood sugars.

For some people, other issues may be contributing to poor eating habits and weight gain. These may be due to long working hours, family commitments, shift work or travelling. Disrupted or inadequate sleep, or prolonged and excessive stress can also make it harder. But by making helpful lifestyle changes you start to feel better and can get into a positive cycle.

On the next page you can think about and record what you want to achieve with the Fast 800 and I hope you enjoy the recipes that food writer Justine Pattison and I have put together. And thank you to my niece Emily Mosley for the lovely drawings. You can also find recipe photos at www.thefast800.com to inspire you.

Dr Clare Bailey

WHAT DIFFERENCE WILL DOING THE FAST 800 MAKE TO YOU?
HOW WILL YOU KNOW WHEN YOU HAVE REACHED YOUR GOAL?

HOW IMPORTANT IS IT TO YOU?

1   2   3   4   5   6   7   8   9   10

WHAT COULD GET IN YOUR WAY?

WHAT COULD YOU DO TO REDUCE THIS?
WHO COULD HELP SUPPORT YOU?

What specific targets are you aiming for?

	CURRENT	TARGET
WEIGHT		
BMI (*see footnote)		
WAIST		
HbA1C (**)		
OTHER		

* BMI a measure of whether you are a healthy weight for your height
(see https://patient.info/doctor/bmi-calculator-calculator)
** This is an optional blood test that gives you the average
of your recent blood sugar levels over 2-3 months

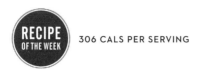

306 CALS PER SERVING

Baked mozzarella fritters

These low-carb cheesy fritters have a Mediterranean flavour and are ideal as a light meal. Serve with a large salad (add calories for dressing) or they are good eaten cold for lunch on the go.

SERVES 2
2 medium eggs
300g cauliflower florets, coarsely grated
½ tsp dried oregano
125g ready-grated mozzarella

1. Preheat the oven to 220°C/fan 200°C/Gas 7. Line a large baking tray with non-stick baking paper.

2. Crack the eggs into a large bowl and whisk until smooth. Add the cauliflower, oregano and 75g of the mozzarella. Season with a good pinch of salt and lots of ground black pepper.

3. Spoon the cauliflower mixture on to the lined tray in six heaps, spacing them well apart. Press down slightly with a spatula or the back of a spoon then bake for about 15 minutes, or until golden and crisp around the edges.

4. Take the tray out of the oven, sprinkle fritters with the remaining mozzarella and bake for a further 5 minutes, or until the cheese has melted and is beginning to bubble.

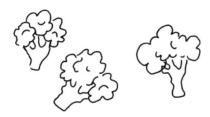

Week One
TARGETS & AIMS

WRITE DOWN YOUR WEIGHT

ANY BIG EVENTS OR OCCASIONS YOU NEED TO FACTOR IN?

WHAT ARE YOUR GOALS THIS WEEK?

WHICH WILL BE YOUR FASTING DAYS?

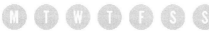

Remember: small steps, big change...

FOOD PLANNER

Plan your meals for the week ahead

	MONDAY	TUESDAY	WEDNESDAY	THURSDAY
BREAKFAST				
LUNCH				
DINNER				
(SNACK)				
CALORIES				

FRIDAY	SATURDAY	SUNDAY	
			TOTAL CALORIES

SHOPPING LIST

NOTES

Week One
MONDAY

BREAKFAST	CALORIES

LUNCH	

DINNER	

(SNACK)	

TOTAL

TRE	WATER	MOOD	SLEEP
10 12 14	◯ ◑ ●	☺ ☺ ☹	☺ ☺ ☹

ACTIVITY

WHAT WORKED?

Week One
TUESDAY

BREAKFAST	CALORIES
LUNCH	
DINNER	
(SNACK)	
	TOTAL

TRE	WATER	MOOD	SLEEP
10 12 14	◯ ◑ ●	🙂 😐 🙁	🙂 😐 🙁

ACTIVITY

WHAT WORKED?

23

Week One
WEDNESDAY

NON-FASTING DAY   800 DAY

BREAKFAST	CALORIES
LUNCH	
DINNER	
(SNACK)	

TOTAL

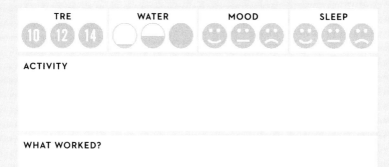

TRE   WATER   MOOD   SLEEP

10 12 14

ACTIVITY

WHAT WORKED?

Week One
THURSDAY

NON-FASTING DAY   800 DAY

	CALORIES
BREAKFAST	
LUNCH	
DINNER	
(SNACK)	
	TOTAL

TRE	WATER	MOOD	SLEEP
10 12 14	◯ ◑ ◉	🙂 😐 🙁	🙂 😐 🙁

ACTIVITY

WHAT WORKED?

25

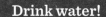

Drink water!

We cannot stress this often
enough... Keeping well hydrated is
vital for maintaining energy levels
and helping to reduce hunger pangs.
Most people need an extra 1–1½ litres
of water on 800 days, when they are
fasting, as they are not only missing
out on the fluid they would normally
get in their meals, but also losing
water in the process of burning fat.
Don't wait till you feel thirsty.
Try and stay ahead of the game.

Week One
FRIDAY

NON-FASTING DAY   800 DAY

	CALORIES
BREAKFAST	
LUNCH	
DINNER	
(SNACK)	
	TOTAL

TRE	WATER	MOOD	SLEEP
10 12 14			

ACTIVITY

WHAT WORKED?

Week One
SATURDAY

NON-FASTING DAY ○   800 DAY ○

BREAKFAST	CALORIES

LUNCH	

DINNER	

(SNACK)	

	TOTAL

TRE	WATER	MOOD	SLEEP

ACTIVITY

WHAT WORKED?

Week One
SUNDAY

NON-FASTING DAY   800 DAY

BREAKFAST	CALORIES
LUNCH	
DINNER	
(SNACK)	
	TOTAL

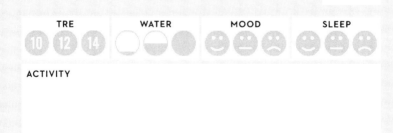

TRE   WATER   MOOD   SLEEP

ACTIVITY

WHAT WORKED?

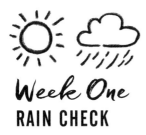

Week One
RAIN CHECK

The first few weeks on Stage 1 of the Fast 800 are usually the most challenging, whilst your body adapts. You can choose to eat two or three meals a day but aim to stick to around 800 calories.

The fastest weight loss generally occurs in weeks one and two, along with fluid loss. Remember to keep well hydrated, drinking at least 1–1½ litres of water a day. Some may find it helpful to use meal replacement shakes for some meals at this stage, e.g. for breakfast or to take to work at lunch. Choose good-quality, low-carb versions with adequate protein. You can record these in the journal, too.

Those of you who don't have much weight to lose or who are not suited to 800-calorie fasting may choose to go straight to Stage 2 (the New 5:2).

Whatever plan you are following, it's important to try and avoid snacking between meals as it stops fat-burning.

"There are so many people all over the world with the same weight and eating habits as mine. I tended to think I was the only overweight person in the village. Being able to change from Fast 800 to the New 5:2 or Mediterranean diet was also very welcome." Valerie

WEIGHT	NUMBER OF 800 DAYS THIS WEEK
WAIST	NUMBER OF NON-FASTING DAYS THIS WEEK

FOOD: WHAT WORKED AND WHAT DO YOU PLAN TO CHANGE?

ACTIVITY: WHAT WORKED AND WHAT DO YOU PLAN TO CHANGE?

WATER INTAKE	OVERALL MOOD	OVERALL SLEEP

HOW ARE YOU COPING AND WHAT DO YOU PLAN TO CHANGE?

WHAT ARE YOU MOST PROUD OF?

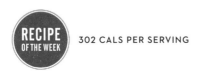

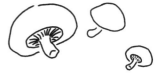

Beef and mushroom casserole

Serve with a generous portion of freshly cooked kale or shredded cabbage, with insignificant added calories. Mashed celeriac or swede would also go well, but don't forget to add the extra calories.

SERVES 4
450g braising or stewing steak, trimmed
    and cut into roughly 2.5cm chunks
3 tbsp olive oil
1 medium onion, peeled and thinly sliced
3 celery sticks, cut into roughly 1.5cm slices
2 large carrots (around 300g), trimmed, halved
    lengthways and cut into roughly 1.5cm slices
250g small mushrooms, halved
1 beef stock cube
2 tbsp tomato purée
1 tsp dried mixed herbs

1. Preheat the oven to 170°C/fan 150°C/Gas 3. Season the beef all over with salt and freshly ground black pepper.

2. Heat 1 tablespoon of the oil in a large non-stick frying pan and fry the beef in batches over a medium-high heat for 2–3 minutes, or until browned. Transfer to a flame-proof casserole dish.

3. Add the remaining oil to the frying pan and cook the onion, celery, carrots and mushrooms for 5 minutes, or until lightly browned, stirring regularly. You may need to do this in batches. Add to the casserole dish.

4. Crumble over the stock cube and stir in the tomato purée and 450ml cold water. Sprinkle with the herbs and bring to a simmer, stirring occasionally.

5. Cover with a lid and place in the oven to cook for about 2 hours, or until the beef is very tender.

Week Two
TARGETS & AIMS

WRITE DOWN YOUR WEIGHT

ANY BIG EVENTS OR OCCASIONS YOU NEED TO FACTOR IN?

WHAT ARE YOUR GOALS THIS WEEK?

WHICH WILL BE YOUR FASTING DAYS?

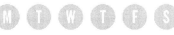

The time for action is now. It's never too late to do something. *The Little Prince*

FOOD PLANNER

Plan your meals for the week ahead

	MONDAY	TUESDAY	WEDNESDAY	THURSDAY
BREAKFAST				
LUNCH				
DINNER				
(SNACK)				
CALORIES				

FRIDAY	SATURDAY	SUNDAY	
			TOTAL CALORIES

SHOPPING LIST

NOTES

Week Two
MONDAY

NON-FASTING DAY   800 DAY

BREAKFAST	CALORIES

LUNCH	

DINNER	

(SNACK)	

TOTAL

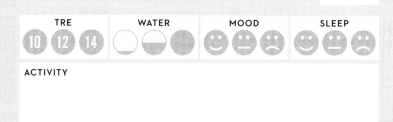

TRE	WATER	MOOD	SLEEP
10 12 14			

ACTIVITY

WHAT WORKED?

Week Two
TUESDAY

BREAKFAST	CALORIES
LUNCH	
DINNER	
(SNACK)	
	TOTAL

TRE	WATER	MOOD	SLEEP
10 12 14			

ACTIVITY

WHAT WORKED?

Week Two
WEDNESDAY

NON-FASTING DAY   800 DAY

BREAKFAST	CALORIES
LUNCH	
DINNER	
(SNACK)	
	TOTAL

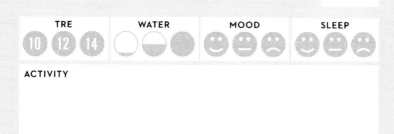

TRE   10 12 14

WATER

MOOD

SLEEP

ACTIVITY

WHAT WORKED?

Week Two
THURSDAY

○ NON-FASTING DAY   ○ 800 DAY

BREAKFAST	CALORIES

LUNCH	

DINNER	

(SNACK)	

	TOTAL

TRE	WATER	MOOD	SLEEP
10 12 14	○ ◐ ●	☺ ☺ ☹	☺ ☺ ☹

ACTIVITY

WHAT WORKED?

Find a fasting friend.

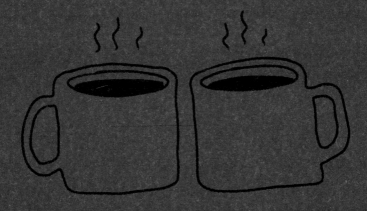

Being part of a group – even if it's just you and a friend – will significantly improve your chances of success. It is also vital that people close to you understand why you are doing this diet and what you want to achieve. So tell your friends and family about it and that you need them to be supportive – i.e. not encouraging you to have a piece of cake with your coffee.

Week Two
FRIDAY

BREAKFAST	CALORIES

LUNCH	

DINNER	

(SNACK)	

	TOTAL

TRE	WATER	MOOD	SLEEP

ACTIVITY

WHAT WORKED?

Week Two
SATURDAY

NON-FASTING DAY   800 DAY

BREAKFAST	CALORIES

LUNCH	

DINNER	

(SNACK)	

	TOTAL

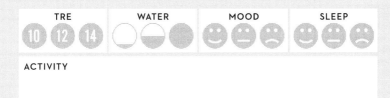

TRE   WATER   MOOD   SLEEP

ACTIVITY

WHAT WORKED?

Week Two
SUNDAY

NON-FASTING DAY   800 DAY

	CALORIES
BREAKFAST	
LUNCH	
DINNER	
(SNACK)	
TOTAL	

TRE	WATER	MOOD	SLEEP
10 12 14	⬤ ⬤ ⬤	🙂 😐 ☹️	🙂 😐 ☹️

ACTIVITY

WHAT WORKED?

END OF WEEK 2 REVIEW

Well done! It usually gets easier from here. If your blood sugar or blood pressure has been raised, you may see a reduction now. You might wish to check in with your health professional at this point for a review. This is also a good time to start to increase your activity levels.

You may find your appetite is under better control and you are feeling more energetic. Rapid weight loss is very motivating. Evidence shows that people who lose weight fast tend to lose more fat and to keep it off long term. So if you have more to lose, try to stick with the Fast 800 days.

If, however, you are finding 800 calories too tough, you might want to add a few non-fasting days, perhaps at weekends, or move to the New 5:2 or even to the Fast 800 Way of Life – i.e. where you stick to a lowish carb Med-style diet, no longer counting calories but being careful about your portion size.

And don't forget to check your "kitchen hygiene" to make it easier for you – put temptations out of sight or ideally remove them altogether!

"It was so much easier than I thought it would be!" Marion

WAIST

WEIGHT

HOW ARE YOU COPING EMOTIONALLY AND PHYSICALLY?
TIME TO REVIEW THE NUMBER OF 800 CAL DAYS?

WHAT DIFFERENCE IS THIS DIET MAKING?
WHAT ARE THE CHANGES?

HOW IMPORTANT IS YOUR GOAL?

① ② ③ ④ ⑤ ⑥ ⑦ ⑧ ⑨ ⑩

HOW CONFIDENT ARE YOU THAT YOU WILL REACH YOUR GOAL?

① ② ③ ④ ⑤ ⑥ ⑦ ⑧ ⑨ ⑩

WHAT WORKS? HOW COULD YOU INCREASE THE LIKELIHOOD
THAT YOU REACH YOUR GOAL?

WHAT ARE YOU MOST PROUD OF?

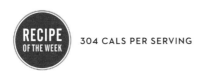

304 CALS PER SERVING

Chicken and chorizo pilaf

A delicious dish that includes some healthy complex carbs, in the form of bulgur wheat, that are good for your microbiome – those helpful bugs in your gut.

SERVES 4
1 tbsp olive oil
4 boneless, skinless chicken thighs (around 400g), trimmed and cut into roughly 1.5cm slices
1 large onion, peeled and finely chopped
150g mushrooms (any kind), sliced
50g chorizo sausage, diced
100g bulgur wheat
500ml chicken stock (made using 1 chicken stock cube)
small bunch parsley, roughly chopped (optional)
large portion of green beans, kale, cabbage or spinach, to serve

1. Heat the oil in a wide-based casserole or large deep frying pan. Add the chicken and onion and fry gently for 5 minutes, or until the onion is softened, stirring regularly.

2. Increase the heat, add the mushrooms and chorizo and cook for 3 minutes, stirring constantly.

3. Add the bulgur wheat and chicken stock, season with lots of ground black pepper and bring to a gentle simmer.

4. Reduce the heat and cook for about 15 minutes, or until the bulgur wheat is tender and almost all the liquid has been absorbed, stirring regularly. Add an extra splash of water if needed.

5. Sprinkle with parsley, if using, and serve with large portions of freshly cooked green vegetables.

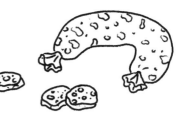

Week Three
TARGETS & AIMS

WRITE DOWN YOUR WEIGHT

ANY BIG EVENTS OR OCCASIONS YOU NEED TO FACTOR IN?

WHAT ARE YOUR GOALS THIS WEEK?

WHICH WILL BE YOUR FASTING DAYS?

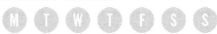

Instead of focusing on circumstances you can't change – focus on those you can.

FOOD PLANNER

Plan your meals for the week ahead

	MONDAY	TUESDAY	WEDNESDAY	THURSDAY
BREAKFAST				
LUNCH				
DINNER				
(SNACK)				
CALORIES				

FRIDAY	SATURDAY	SUNDAY	
			TOTAL CALORIES

SHOPPING LIST

NOTES

Week Three
MONDAY

○ NON-FASTING DAY   ○ 800 DAY

BREAKFAST	CALORIES

LUNCH	

DINNER	

(SNACK)	

TOTAL

TRE	WATER	MOOD	SLEEP
10 12 14	◯ ◑ ●	☺ ☺ ☹	☺ 😐 ☹

ACTIVITY

WHAT WORKED?

Week Three
TUESDAY

BREAKFAST	CALORIES
LUNCH	
DINNER	
(SNACK)	
	TOTAL

TRE	WATER	MOOD	SLEEP
10 12 14			

ACTIVITY

WHAT WORKED?

Week Three
WEDNESDAY

NON-FASTING DAY   800 DAY

BREAKFAST	CALORIES
LUNCH	
DINNER	
(SNACK)	
	TOTAL

TRE	WATER	MOOD	SLEEP
10 12 14	◯ ◖ ●	😊 😐 ☹	😊 😐 ☹

ACTIVITY

WHAT WORKED?

56

Week Three
THURSDAY

BREAKFAST

CALORIES

LUNCH

DINNER

(SNACK)

TOTAL

TRE	WATER	MOOD	SLEEP
10 12 14	◯ ◑ ●	☺ 😐 ☹	☺ 😐 ☹

ACTIVITY

WHAT WORKED?

Ten healthy foods to keep on your shopping list:

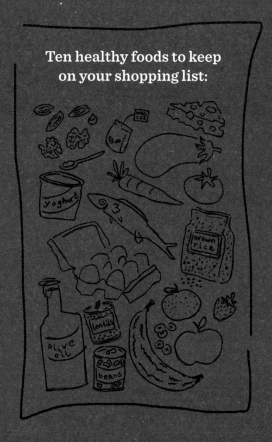

Olive oil, non-starchy vegetables, full-fat yoghurt and cheese, unsalted nuts, wholegrains such as brown rice or quinoa, eggs, oily fish, beans and lentils, fizzy water and herbal teas.

Week Three
FRIDAY

NON-FASTING DAY   800 DAY

BREAKFAST	CALORIES

LUNCH	

DINNER	

(SNACK)	

TOTAL

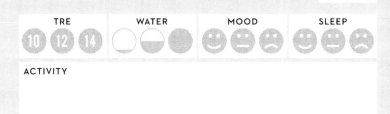

TRE   10   12   14   WATER   MOOD   SLEEP

ACTIVITY

WHAT WORKED?

Week Three
SATURDAY

BREAKFAST	CALORIES

LUNCH	

DINNER	

(SNACK)	

	TOTAL

TRE	WATER	MOOD	SLEEP
10 12 14			

ACTIVITY

WHAT WORKED?

60

Week Three
SUNDAY

BREAKFAST	CALORIES
LUNCH	
DINNER	
(SNACK)	
	TOTAL

TRE	WATER	MOOD	SLEEP
10 12 14	○ ◑ ●	😊 😐 ☹️	😊 😐 ☹️

ACTIVITY

WHAT WORKED?

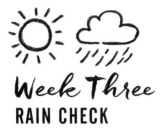

Week Three
RAIN CHECK

By now you should have cut right back on sweet and starchy processed carbs, including bread, potatoes, white rice, processed cereals and white pasta, and hopefully your taste buds will have adjusted so that you are no longer missing them as much. Remember the key to avoiding temptation is to plan well ahead. Use the weekly food planner and do try the simple, low-carb recipes in this journal. For more options go to www.thefast800.com.

Have you added in Time Restricted Eating (TRE) yet? This is where you eat within a narrower time window to increase the length of your overnight fast. Start with 12:12, which means eating within a 12-hour period and not later than three hours before you sleep.

"From someone who has always struggled with being 'hangry', miraculously, this will no longer affect you. No or little willpower required!" Bridget

WEIGHT	NUMBER OF 800 DAYS THIS WEEK
WAIST	NUMBER OF NON-FASTING DAYS THIS WEEK

FOOD: WHAT WORKED AND WHAT DO YOU PLAN TO CHANGE?

ACTIVITY: WHAT WORKED AND WHAT DO YOU PLAN TO CHANGE?

WATER INTAKE	OVERALL MOOD	OVERALL SLEEP

HOW ARE YOU COPING AND WHAT DO YOU PLAN TO CHANGE?

WHAT ARE YOU MOST PROUD OF?

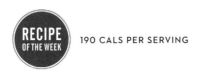
Date & pecan baked apples

A quick and easy upside-down baked apple dish. Delicious served hot or cold. Serve with full-fat live Greek yoghurt, if you like, but don't forget to add the extra calories.

SERVES 4
5g coconut oil, for greasing
40g soft pitted dates (around 4), chopped
50g pecan nuts, roughly chopped
finely grated zest 1 small lemon
½ tsp ground cinnamon
3 medium cooking apples (around 250g each), quartered and cored

1. Preheat the oven to 200°C/fan 180°C/Gas 6. Grease the base of a roughly 20cm diameter ovenproof dish with the oil.

2. Add the dates, nuts, lemon zest and cinnamon to the dish and toss to mix.

3. Set the apple quarters on top of the fruit and nuts in a single layer, skin-side up. Pack the apples in tightly to cover the dried fruit so it doesn't burn. Pour 5 tablespoons cold water over the top and bake for 25–30 minutes, or until the apples are soft.

COOK'S TIP: You can also cook these apples in the microwave. Assemble as above in a microwave-safe dish and cook on HIGH for 8–9 minutes. (Recipe tested using a 900W microwave oven – you might need to adjust the timing.)

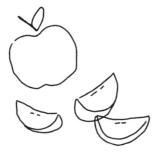

Week Four
TARGETS & AIMS

WRITE DOWN YOUR WEIGHT

ANY BIG EVENTS OR OCCASIONS YOU NEED TO FACTOR IN?

WHAT ARE YOUR GOALS THIS WEEK?

WHICH WILL BE YOUR FASTING DAYS?

(M) (T) (W) (T) (F) (S) (S)

The most effective way to do it, is to do it. *Amelia Earhart*

FOOD PLANNER

Plan your meals for the week ahead

	MONDAY	TUESDAY	WEDNESDAY	THURSDAY
BREAKFAST				
LUNCH				
DINNER				
(SNACK)				
CALORIES				

FRIDAY	SATURDAY	SUNDAY

TOTAL
CALORIES

SHOPPING LIST

NOTES

Week Four
MONDAY

NON-FASTING DAY   800 DAY

BREAKFAST	CALORIES

LUNCH	

DINNER	

(SNACK)	

	TOTAL

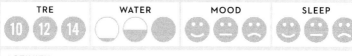

TRE	WATER	MOOD	SLEEP
10 12 14			

ACTIVITY

WHAT WORKED?

Week Four
TUESDAY

BREAKFAST	CALORIES
LUNCH	
DINNER	
(SNACK)	

TOTAL

TRE	WATER	MOOD	SLEEP
10 12 14			

ACTIVITY

WHAT WORKED?

71

Week Four
WEDNESDAY

NON-FASTING DAY   800 DAY

BREAKFAST	CALORIES

LUNCH	

DINNER	

(SNACK)	

TOTAL

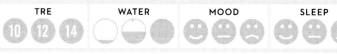

TRE	WATER	MOOD	SLEEP
10 12 14			

ACTIVITY

WHAT WORKED?

Week Four
THURSDAY

NON-FASTING DAY   800 DAY

BREAKFAST	CALORIES

LUNCH	

DINNER	

(SNACK)	

TOTAL

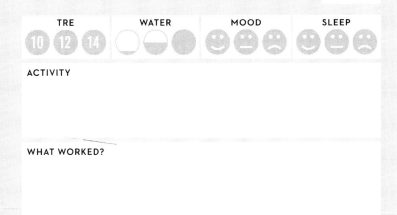

TRE   WATER   MOOD   SLEEP

ACTIVITY

WHAT WORKED?

Always take the stairs. And, if possible, try and run up them.

This is a wonderfully simple way of upping your daily activity and burning calories as you go.

Week Four
FRIDAY

NON-FASTING DAY   800 DAY

BREAKFAST	CALORIES
LUNCH	
DINNER	
(SNACK)	

TOTAL

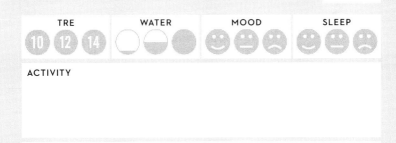

TRE	WATER	MOOD	SLEEP
10 12 14			

ACTIVITY

WHAT WORKED?

Week Four
SATURDAY

NON-FASTING DAY   800 DAY

BREAKFAST	CALORIES

LUNCH	

DINNER	

(SNACK)	

	TOTAL

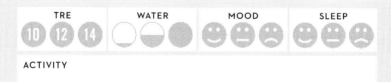

TRE   10   12   14   WATER   MOOD   SLEEP

ACTIVITY

WHAT WORKED?

Week Four
SUNDAY

NON-FASTING DAY   800 DAY

BREAKFAST	CALORIES
LUNCH	
DINNER	
(SNACK)	
	TOTAL

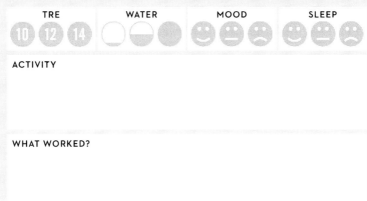

TRE	WATER	MOOD	SLEEP

ACTIVITY

WHAT WORKED?

MONTHLY REVIEW

Excellent! You have now completed four weeks of the Fast 800. Your efforts will have had a significant beneficial impact on your metabolism. By now you should be feeling more energetic, thinking more clearly and be lighter in your step. Your waist will have reduced and you are hopefully increasing your activity levels.

If you have more weight to lose, stick with the 800-calorie days if it's suiting you, as you can continue this for up to 12 weeks if needed. But remember to include plenty of healthy fat, as this will keep you full for longer and help weight loss.

You may be getting close to your goal. If so, you may choose to move to the New 5:2 approach, if you haven't done so already. Or even to the Way of Life, where you eat a low-carb, Mediterranean-style diet with portion control but no longer count calories.

"I've changed my whole lifestyle and, while I still have days that may not go to plan, I can make better choices and return to better habits. I'm more mindful around what I eat, when I eat and I feel healthier." Joanne

WAIST

WEIGHT

HOW ARE YOU COPING EMOTIONALLY AND PHYSICALLY?
TIME TO REVIEW THE NUMBER OF 800 CAL DAYS?
TIME FOR A MEDICATION/HEALTH PROFESSIONAL REVIEW?

WHAT DIFFERENCE IS THIS DIET MAKING?
WHAT ARE THE CHANGES?

HOW IMPORTANT IS YOUR GOAL?

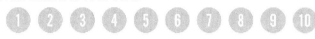

HOW CONFIDENT ARE YOU THAT YOU WILL REACH YOUR GOAL?

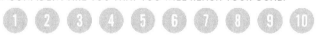

WHAT WORKS? HOW COULD YOU INCREASE THE LIKELIHOOD
THAT YOU REACH YOUR GOAL?

WHAT ARE YOU MOST PROUD OF?

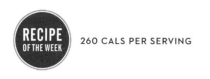 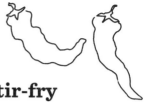

RECIPE OF THE WEEK 260 CALS PER SERVING

Ginger chilli prawn stir-fry

I'm a big fan of stir-fries as quick, flavoursome, one-pan dishes.

SERVES 2

1 tbsp coconut, rapeseed or olive oil
1 red pepper, deseeded and cut into roughly 2.5cm chunks
2 medium carrots, trimmed and thinly sliced (optional)
½ medium onion, peeled and cut into 8 wedges
1 garlic clove, peeled and thinly sliced
20g fresh root ginger, peeled and thinly sliced
100g curly kale, thickly shredded with any tough stalks discarded
1 tsp cornflour
1½ tbsp dark soy sauce
½ tsp dried chilli flakes, or 1 small red chilli, finely sliced
150g cooked and peeled prawns, thawed and drained

For the cauli-rice
200g cauliflower, coarsely grated

1. Place the cauliflower in a microwave-safe bowl, cover and cook on HIGH for 3 minutes, or until tender. For other methods of cooking the cauliflower see page 242 of *The Fast 800 Recipe Book*.

2. Meanwhile, heat the oil in a large non-stick frying pan or wok. Add the pepper, carrots and onion and stir-fry over a medium-high heat for 3–4 minutes.

3. Add the garlic, ginger and kale and cook for a further minute, or until the kale has softened, stirring regularly.

4. Mix the cornflour with the soy sauce and chilli flakes in a small bowl. Add 3 tablespoons cold water and stir until thoroughly combined. Add the sauce and prawns to the pan and toss together for 1 minute or until hot throughout.

COOK'S TIP: Use thinly sliced beef steak or chicken breast instead of the prawns, if you like. Add with the pepper and carrots.

NON-FAST DAY: Enjoy a larger portion or serve with 2–3 tablespoons cooked brown or wild rice or some Japanese Soba noodles.

Week Five
TARGETS & AIMS

WRITE DOWN YOUR WEIGHT

ANY BIG EVENTS OR OCCASIONS YOU NEED TO FACTOR IN?

WHAT ARE YOUR GOALS THIS WEEK?

WHICH WILL BE YOUR FASTING DAYS?

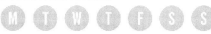

If you've fallen off the wagon, don't despair or give in to catastrophic thinking that you've failed – it happens to most people. Just start again tomorrow...

FOOD PLANNER

Plan your meals for the week ahead

	MONDAY	TUESDAY	WEDNESDAY	THURSDAY
BREAKFAST				
LUNCH				
DINNER				
(SNACK)				
CALORIES				

FRIDAY	SATURDAY	SUNDAY	
			TOTAL CALORIES

SHOPPING LIST

NOTES

Week Five
MONDAY

NON-FASTING DAY ◯   800 DAY ◯

BREAKFAST	CALORIES

LUNCH	

DINNER	

(SNACK)	

	TOTAL

TRE	WATER	MOOD	SLEEP
10 12 14	◯ ◑ ●	☺ ☹	☺ ☹

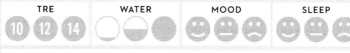

ACTIVITY

WHAT WORKED?

Week Five
TUESDAY

○ NON-FASTING DAY   ○ 800 DAY

BREAKFAST	CALORIES

LUNCH	

DINNER	

(SNACK)	

TOTAL

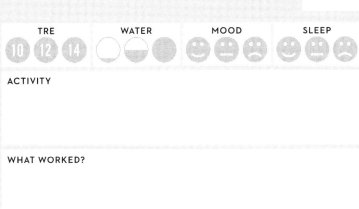

TRE 10 12 14

WATER

MOOD

SLEEP

ACTIVITY

WHAT WORKED?

Week Five
WEDNESDAY

BREAKFAST	CALORIES

LUNCH	

DINNER	

(SNACK)	

	TOTAL

TRE	WATER	MOOD	SLEEP
10 12 14			

ACTIVITY

WHAT WORKED?

Week Five
THURSDAY

NON-FASTING DAY   800 DAY

	CALORIES
BREAKFAST	
LUNCH	
DINNER	
(SNACK)	
	TOTAL

TRE	WATER	MOOD	SLEEP
10 12 14			

ACTIVITY

WHAT WORKED?

Make soup.

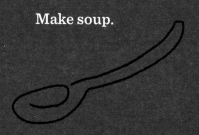

It is satiating, cheap, practical and highly nutritious. You can make it in big quantities – it's a great way of using up leftover veg – and keep any extras in the fridge or freezer.

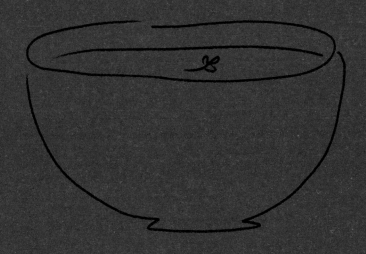

Week Five
FRIDAY

BREAKFAST	CALORIES

LUNCH	

DINNER	

(SNACK)	

TOTAL

TRE	WATER	MOOD	SLEEP
10 12 14			

ACTIVITY

WHAT WORKED?

Week Five
SATURDAY

NON-FASTING DAY　　800 DAY

BREAKFAST	CALORIES
LUNCH	
DINNER	
(SNACK)	
	TOTAL

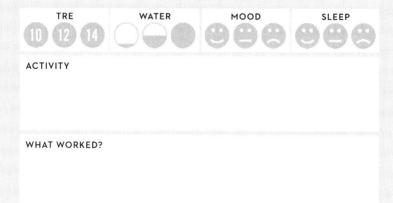

TRE
10 12 14

WATER

MOOD

SLEEP

ACTIVITY

WHAT WORKED?

Week Five
SUNDAY

NON-FASTING DAY   800 DAY

BREAKFAST	CALORIES

LUNCH	

DINNER	

(SNACK)	

TOTAL

TRE	WATER	MOOD	SLEEP
10 12 14			

ACTIVITY

WHAT WORKED?

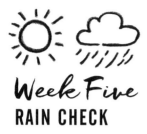

Week Five
RAIN CHECK

To enhance the effect, you can reduce your eating window further by moving on to a 14:10 TRE (Time Restricted Eating) approach. This means eating within a 10-hour window, increasing your overnight fast to 14 hours.

Studies on mice have shown that eating within a restricted period can have a dramatic impact on weight loss. But it's not just about shedding the pounds. "Time-restricted eating" has been used in religious practice for centuries. More than 2500 years ago Buddha told his followers that, if they made it their practice to stop eating after their midday meal and fast until the following morning, they would achieve enhanced mental clarity and a sense of wellbeing.

"A lot of 'a-ha' moments, especially TRE. Eating full-fat food surprised me, too, after eating low fat most of my life. The taste is so different and I won't be going back to low fat and the chemical additives to make up for taste." Valerie

WEIGHT	NUMBER OF 800 DAYS THIS WEEK
WAIST	NUMBER OF NON-FASTING DAYS THIS WEEK

FOOD: WHAT WORKED AND WHAT DO YOU PLAN TO CHANGE?

ACTIVITY: WHAT WORKED AND WHAT DO YOU PLAN TO CHANGE?

WATER INTAKE	OVERALL MOOD	OVERALL SLEEP

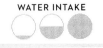

HOW ARE YOU COPING AND WHAT DO YOU PLAN TO CHANGE?

WHAT ARE YOU MOST PROUD OF?

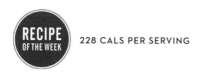

RECIPE OF THE WEEK

High protein nutty chocolate shake

Maintaining adequate protein, whilst staying low carb, can
be a challenge on 800 calories, particularly for vegetarians.
This delicious protein shake will help maintain your daily
protein requirement (around 50–60g per day).

SERVES 1
1 tbsp no-added-sugar almond or cashew
    nut butter (around 15g)
4g cocoa powder (around 2 tsp)
6g organic whey powder (around 1 tbsp)
150ml full-fat milk

1. Put all the ingredients in a blender and blitz until smooth.

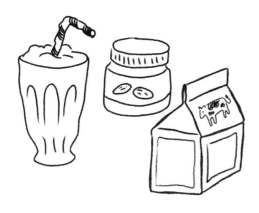

Week Six
TARGETS & AIMS

WRITE DOWN YOUR WEIGHT

ANY BIG EVENTS OR OCCASIONS YOU NEED TO FACTOR IN?

WHAT ARE YOUR GOALS THIS WEEK?

WHICH WILL BE YOUR FASTING DAYS?

Remember to check in with your friends.

FOOD PLANNER

Plan your meals for the week ahead

	MONDAY	TUESDAY	WEDNESDAY	THURSDAY
BREAKFAST				
LUNCH				
DINNER				
(SNACK)				
CALORIES				

FRIDAY	SATURDAY	SUNDAY	
			TOTAL CALORIES

SHOPPING LIST

NOTES

Week Six
MONDAY

○ NON-FASTING DAY   ○ 800 DAY

BREAKFAST	CALORIES

LUNCH	

DINNER	

(SNACK)	

	TOTAL

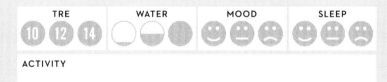

TRE	WATER	MOOD	SLEEP
10 12 14	○ ◐ ●	😊 😐 ☹	😊 😐 ☹

ACTIVITY

WHAT WORKED?

NON-FASTING DAY   800 DAY

BREAKFAST	CALORIES

LUNCH	

DINNER	

(SNACK)	

TOTAL

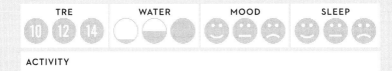

TRE   WATER   MOOD   SLEEP

ACTIVITY

WHAT WORKED?

Week Six
WEDNESDAY

NON-FASTING DAY   800 DAY

BREAKFAST	CALORIES

LUNCH	

DINNER	

(SNACK)	

TOTAL

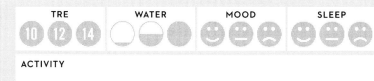

TRE   10 12 14

WATER

MOOD

SLEEP

ACTIVITY

WHAT WORKED?

Week Six
THURSDAY

BREAKFAST	CALORIES

LUNCH	

DINNER	

(SNACK)	

TOTAL

TRE	WATER	MOOD	SLEEP
10 12 14	○ ◐ ●	😊 😐 ☹️	😊 😐 ☹️

ACTIVITY

WHAT WORKED?

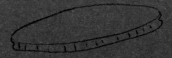

Plan ahead if you are going to be
out all day or working shifts.

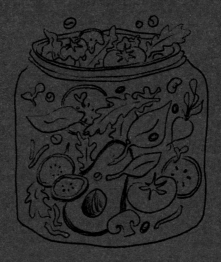

Making and taking your lunch to work
is not only healthier, but cheaper too.
Much better than dropping into
the nearest sandwich bar!

Take soup or leftovers in a container.
Assemble a salad in a jar. If you can't
keep it cool, assemble it in a bowl
from small tins and a small bottle
of dressing – cannellini beans and
tuna works well. Be creative!

Week Six
FRIDAY

○ NON-FASTING DAY   ○ 800 DAY

BREAKFAST	CALORIES

LUNCH	

DINNER	

(SNACK)	

	TOTAL

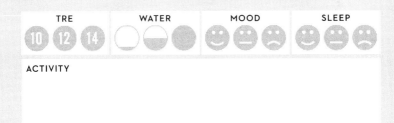

TRE	WATER	MOOD	SLEEP
10 12 14	○ ◐ ●	😊 😐 ☹️	😊 😐 ☹️

ACTIVITY

WHAT WORKED?

Week Six
SATURDAY

NON-FASTING DAY   800 DAY

BREAKFAST	CALORIES

LUNCH	

DINNER	

(SNACK)	

	TOTAL

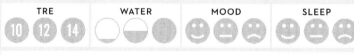

TRE	WATER	MOOD	SLEEP
10 12 14			

ACTIVITY

WHAT WORKED?

Week Six
SUNDAY

NON-FASTING DAY   800 DAY

BREAKFAST	CALORIES
LUNCH	
DINNER	
(SNACK)	

TOTAL

TRE	WATER	MOOD	SLEEP
10 12 14			

ACTIVITY

WHAT WORKED?

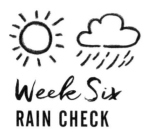

Week Six
RAIN CHECK

Some people experience a temporary weight loss plateau around this time. Review what you are doing to make sure you are following the programme and that portions haven't crept up again! Try to build more activity into your day. Take the stairs, add a bike ride to your day, or perhaps get off the bus a couple of stops early and walk the last stretch. But remember, the most important thing is to try and move regularly throughout the day. An hour of hard exercise in the gym once or twice a week cannot compensate for sitting at a desk for a full five days.

Are you beginning to enjoy your non-starchy vegetables? They are key to success, so we don't ask you to count the calories for most green and coloured leafy vegetables. Fill half your plate with these.

"I decided to try one last time before I turned myself over to medical science as a phenomenon and, frankly, had very low expectations that this plan would work. That was 12 weeks and 30+ pounds ago." Nancy

WEIGHT	NUMBER OF 800 DAYS THIS WEEK
WAIST	NUMBER OF NON-FASTING DAYS THIS WEEK

FOOD: WHAT WORKED AND WHAT DO YOU PLAN TO CHANGE?

ACTIVITY: WHAT WORKED AND WHAT DO YOU PLAN TO CHANGE?

WATER INTAKE	OVERALL MOOD	OVERALL SLEEP
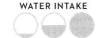		

HOW ARE YOU COPING AND WHAT DO YOU PLAN TO CHANGE?

WHAT ARE YOU MOST PROUD OF?

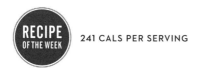

Nutty granola

An indulgent granola that will power you well into your day. A daily portion of nuts has also been shown to reduce heart disease.

SERVES 8
4 tbsp coconut oil
1 tbsp maple syrup
½ tsp ground cinnamon
200g jumbo porridge oats
100g mixed nuts, roughly chopped
15g flaked coconut/coconut chips (optional)

1. Preheat the oven to 170°C/fan 150°C/Gas 3.

2. Melt the coconut oil with the maple syrup and cinnamon in a large saucepan, stirring, over a gentle heat.

3. Remove from the heat and add the oats, stirring until thoroughly mixed. Scatter evenly over a baking tray and bake for 15 minutes.

4. Remove from the oven and stir in the nuts and coconut, if using. Return to the oven for a further 10 minutes.

5. Leave to cool and crisp up on the tray. Store in an airtight jar for up to 2 weeks.

COOK'S TIPS: Serve with around 75ml full-fat milk per 45g portion for an additional 289 calories. Or sprinkle over yoghurt instead, but remember to adjust the calories.

If using flaked coconut, add an extra 10 calories to each serving.

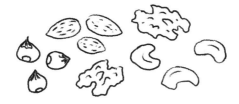

Week Seven
TARGETS & AIMS

WRITE DOWN YOUR WEIGHT

ANY BIG EVENTS OR OCCASIONS YOU NEED TO FACTOR IN?

WHAT ARE YOUR GOALS THIS WEEK?

WHICH WILL BE YOUR FASTING DAYS?

Remember that weight loss is rarely a continuous process: you may plateau, but persist and you will get there.

FOOD PLANNER

Plan your meals for the week ahead

	MONDAY	TUESDAY	WEDNESDAY	THURSDAY
BREAKFAST				
LUNCH				
DINNER				
(SNACK)				
CALORIES				

FRIDAY	SATURDAY	SUNDAY	
			TOTAL CALORIES

SHOPPING LIST

NOTES

Week Seven
MONDAY

NON-FASTING DAY   800 DAY

BREAKFAST	CALORIES
LUNCH	
DINNER	
(SNACK)	
	TOTAL

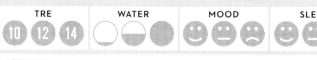

TRE	WATER	MOOD	SLEEP
10 12 14			

ACTIVITY

WHAT WORKED?

Week Seven
TUESDAY

NON-FASTING DAY   800 DAY

BREAKFAST	CALORIES

LUNCH	

DINNER	

(SNACK)	

TOTAL

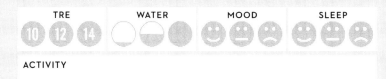

TRE	WATER	MOOD	SLEEP
10 12 14			

ACTIVITY

WHAT WORKED?

Week Seven
WEDNESDAY

NON-FASTING DAY   800 DAY

BREAKFAST	CALORIES

LUNCH	

DINNER	

(SNACK)	

TOTAL

TRE	WATER	MOOD	SLEEP
10 12 14	○ ◐ ●	☺ 😐 ☹	☺ 😐 ☹

ACTIVITY

WHAT WORKED?

Week Seven
THURSDAY

BREAKFAST	CALORIES

LUNCH	

DINNER	

(SNACK)	

TOTAL

TRE	WATER	MOOD	SLEEP
10 12 14	⬤ ⬤ ⬤	☺ 😐 ☹	☺ 😐 ☹

ACTIVITY

WHAT WORKED?

Always try to sit at the table for meals.

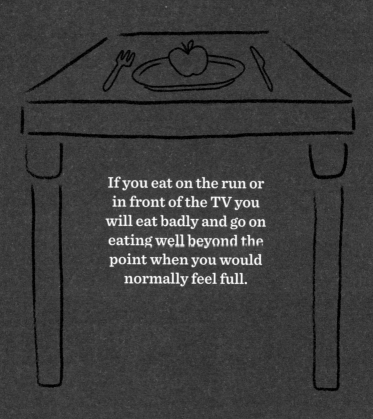

If you eat on the run or
in front of the TV you
will eat badly and go on
eating well beyond the
point when you would
normally feel full.

Week Seven
FRIDAY

NON-FASTING DAY   800 DAY

	CALORIES
BREAKFAST	
LUNCH	
DINNER	
(SNACK)	

	TOTAL

TRE	WATER	MOOD	SLEEP
10 12 14			

ACTIVITY

WHAT WORKED?

Week Seven
SATURDAY

NON-FASTING DAY   800 DAY

BREAKFAST	CALORIES

LUNCH	

DINNER	

(SNACK)	

TOTAL

TRE
10 12 14

WATER

MOOD

SLEEP

ACTIVITY

WHAT WORKED?

Week Seven
SUNDAY

BREAKFAST	CALORIES
LUNCH	
DINNER	
(SNACK)	
	TOTAL

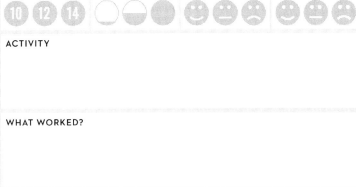

TRE   WATER   MOOD   SLEEP

ACTIVITY

WHAT WORKED?

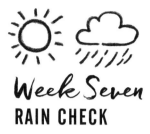

Week Seven
RAIN CHECK

By now you should find that your cravings are really reducing. If you are still finding life without starchy foods a challenge, revisit your goals and remind yourself why you are doing the diet. Distract yourself, call on your back-up support or do something different until it passes – and it will pass! Stay resolute...

"At my last check in with the diabetic nurse, my Hba1c reading was down to 51 from 112, which was after 8 weeks and the nurse was flabbergasted! She couldn't believe it and was totally astounded when I got on the scales." Dermott

WEIGHT	NUMBER OF 800 DAYS THIS WEEK
WAIST	NUMBER OF NON-FASTING DAYS THIS WEEK

FOOD: WHAT WORKED AND WHAT DO YOU PLAN TO CHANGE?

ACTIVITY: WHAT WORKED AND WHAT DO YOU PLAN TO CHANGE?

WATER INTAKE	OVERALL MOOD	OVERALL SLEEP
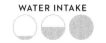		

HOW ARE YOU COPING AND WHAT DO YOU PLAN TO CHANGE?

WHAT ARE YOU MOST PROUD OF?

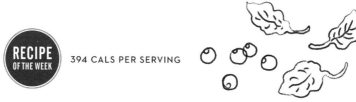

394 CALS PER SERVING

Poached fish with peas & spinach

So easy to cook. We keep white fish, peas and spinach in the freezer, so they are readily at hand for this delicious one-pan dish.

SERVES 2
2 tbsp olive oil
1 medium onion, peeled and finely chopped
3 balls of frozen spinach (around 170g)
150ml stock (made with ½ vegetable or chicken stock cube)
100g frozen peas
finely grated zest ½ small lemon
50g full-fat crème fraîche
2 frozen, skinless white fish fillets,
    such as cod or haddock (each around 100g)

1. Heat the oil in a large lidded frying pan, or wide-based saucepan, and gently fry the onion for 4–5 minutes, or until softened, stirring regularly.

2. Add the frozen spinach and stock, bring to a gentle simmer, then cover with a lid and cook for 5 minutes, or until the spinach is almost thawed.

3. Stir in the peas, lemon zest and crème fraîche. Place the frozen fish fillets on top of the vegetables, season well with ground black pepper, cover with a lid and poach the fish gently for 8–12 minutes, depending on thickness, until the fish is cooked through.

4. Season to taste and serve.

COOK'S TIP: You can make this with fresh spinach and fish but reduce the cooking time accordingly.

NON-FAST DAY: Enjoy a larger portion or serve with 2–3 tablespoons cooked whole grains, such as pearl barley or quinoa, or Puy lentils.

Week Eight
TARGETS & AIMS

WRITE DOWN YOUR WEIGHT

ANY BIG EVENTS OR OCCASIONS YOU NEED TO FACTOR IN?

WHAT ARE YOUR GOALS THIS WEEK?

WHICH WILL BE YOUR FASTING DAYS?

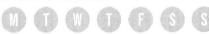

Don't underestimate the importance of getting a good night's sleep!

FOOD PLANNER

Plan your meals for the week ahead

	MONDAY	TUESDAY	WEDNESDAY	THURSDAY
BREAKFAST				
LUNCH				
DINNER				
(SNACK)				
CALORIES				

FRIDAY	SATURDAY	SUNDAY	
			TOTAL CALORIES

SHOPPING LIST

NOTES

Week Eight
MONDAY

○ NON-FASTING DAY   ○ 800 DAY

BREAKFAST	CALORIES

LUNCH	

DINNER	

(SNACK)	

	TOTAL

TRE	WATER	MOOD	SLEEP
10 12 14	○ ◐ ●	😊 😐 ☹️	😊 😐 ☹️

ACTIVITY

WHAT WORKED?

Week Eight
TUESDAY

	CALORIES
BREAKFAST	
LUNCH	
DINNER	
(SNACK)	
	TOTAL

TRE	WATER	MOOD	SLEEP

ACTIVITY

WHAT WORKED?

Week Eight
WEDNESDAY

BREAKFAST	CALORIES

LUNCH	

DINNER	

(SNACK)	

	TOTAL

TRE	WATER	MOOD	SLEEP
10 12 14	○ ◐ ●	😊 😐 ☹️	😊 😐 ☹️

ACTIVITY

WHAT WORKED?

Week Eight
THURSDAY

NON-FASTING DAY   800 DAY

	CALORIES
BREAKFAST	
LUNCH	
DINNER	
(SNACK)	
	TOTAL

TRE	WATER	MOOD	SLEEP
10 12 14	○ ◐ ●	😀 😐 🙁	😀 😐 🙁

ACTIVITY

WHAT WORKED?

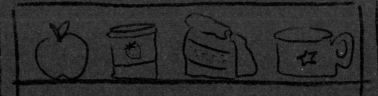

Don't keep your cupboards bare!

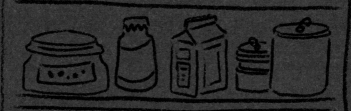

If there is no food in the house you will be much more likely to give in and buy rubbish or order a takeaway. The key to making this diet work is planning. Make sure there is plenty of healthy food around, like nuts, yoghurt and eggs, and keep the fridge stocked with vegetable crudités, such as sticks of carrots, green peppers and cucumber, and perhaps some hummus for moments when you just have to snack.

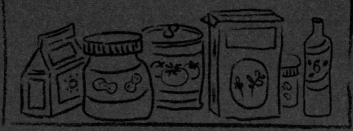

Week Eight
FRIDAY

○ NON-FASTING DAY   ○ 800 DAY

	CALORIES
BREAKFAST	
LUNCH	
DINNER	
(SNACK)	
	TOTAL

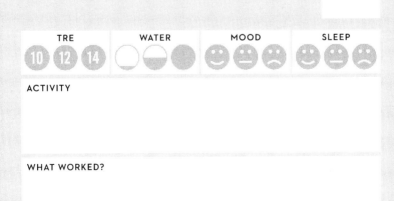

TRE	WATER	MOOD	SLEEP
10 12 14	○ ◓ ●	😀 😐 🙁	😀 😐 🙁

ACTIVITY

WHAT WORKED?

Week Eight
SATURDAY

NON-FASTING DAY   800 DAY

BREAKFAST	CALORIES

LUNCH	

DINNER	

(SNACK)	

	TOTAL

TRE	WATER	MOOD	SLEEP
10 12 14	○ ◐ ●	☺ 😐 ☹	☺ 😐 ☹

ACTIVITY

WHAT WORKED?

140

Week Eight
SUNDAY

BREAKFAST	CALORIES
LUNCH	
DINNER	
(SNACK)	

	TOTAL

TRE	WATER	MOOD	SLEEP
10 12 14	○ ◑ ●	😊 😐 ☹️	😊 😐 ☹️

ACTIVITY

WHAT WORKED?

2nd MONTHLY REVIEW

You are likely to be well on the way by now. If you have remained on the intensive first stage of the Fast 800, keeping to 800 calories daily, you should be seeing significant results and others may be noticing too.

This is a good time to re-evaluate your progress and check in with your health professional if you need to. If you are nearing your goals, you might consider moving to the New 5:2 approach now. If you have reached your goal already – well done! This could be the time to switch to the maintenance stage, where you stick to a low-carb, Med-style diet with portion control and no calorie counting. Either way, celebrate the improvements so far... Hurrah!!

"Very happy with the results – 60 days into the Fast 800 way of eating and I've lost almost 2 stone! If I can do this, anyone can. It doesn't feel like I'm on a diet. Five stars!" Debba

WAIST

WEIGHT

HOW ARE YOU COPING EMOTIONALLY AND PHYSICALLY?
TIME TO REVIEW THE NUMBER OF 800 CAL DAYS?
TIME FOR A MEDICATION/HEALTH PROFESSIONAL REVIEW?

WHAT DIFFERENCE IS THIS DIET MAKING?
WHAT ARE THE CHANGES?

HOW IMPORTANT IS YOUR GOAL?

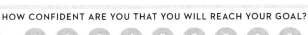

HOW CONFIDENT ARE YOU THAT YOU WILL REACH YOUR GOAL?

WHAT WORKS? HOW COULD YOU INCREASE THE LIKELIHOOD
THAT YOU REACH YOUR GOAL?

WHAT ARE YOU MOST PROUD OF?

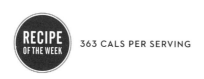
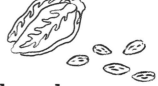

363 CALS PER SERVING

Roast chicory with almonds, apple & blue cheese

This salad is bursting with delicious ingredients that not only taste amazing but also give your microbiome a healthy boost.

SERVES 2
2 tbsp olive oil, plus extra for greasing
2 heads chicory (around 180g each)
25g flaked almonds
2 handfuls mixed salad leaves (around 40g)
1 small red-skinned apple, quartered, cored
    and thinly sliced (90g prepped weight)
½ small lemon

For the dressing
50g soft blue cheese, such as Roquefort
4 tbsp full-fat live Greek yoghurt

1. Preheat the oven to 200°C/fan 180°C/Gas 6. Lightly oil a small baking tray.

2. Trim the chicory and cut in half from root to tip. Place cut-side down in the dish, drizzle over half the oil and bake for 15 minutes.

3. Turn the chicory over and scatter with the almonds. Return to the oven for a further 8–10 minutes, or until the chicory is tender and the almonds are toasted.

4. To make the dressing, place the cheese and yoghurt in a bowl with 3 tablespoons cold water and mash thoroughly with a fork.

5. Divide the chicory and almonds between two plates. Toss the mixed leaves lightly with the remaining oil and place alongside the chicory with the sliced apple. Drizzle everything with the blue cheese dressing, squeeze over the lemon juice and serve.

COOK'S TIP: You can use ½ small cabbage instead of chicory. Cut into 4 lengthways and cook for 25 minutes in step 2. Continue as above.

Week Nine
TARGETS & AIMS

WRITE DOWN YOUR WEIGHT

ANY BIG EVENTS OR OCCASIONS YOU NEED TO FACTOR IN?

WHAT ARE YOUR GOALS THIS WEEK?

WHICH WILL BE YOUR FASTING DAYS?

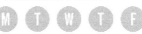

Things do not change; we change. *Henry David Thoreau*

FOOD PLANNER

Plan your meals for the week ahead

	MONDAY	TUESDAY	WEDNESDAY	THURSDAY
BREAKFAST				
LUNCH				
DINNER				
(SNACK)				
CALORIES				

FRIDAY	SATURDAY	SUNDAY	
			TOTAL CALORIES

SHOPPING LIST

NOTES

Week Nine
MONDAY

○ NON-FASTING DAY   ○ 800 DAY

BREAKFAST	CALORIES

LUNCH	

DINNER	

(SNACK)	

	TOTAL

TRE	WATER	MOOD	SLEEP
10 12 14	○ ◐ ●	😊 😐 ☹	😊 😐 ☹

ACTIVITY

WHAT WORKED?

Week Nine
TUESDAY

BREAKFAST	CALORIES

LUNCH	

DINNER	

(SNACK)	

TOTAL

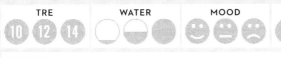

TRE   WATER   MOOD   SLEEP

ACTIVITY

WHAT WORKED?

151

Week Nine
WEDNESDAY

NON-FASTING DAY   800 DAY

BREAKFAST	CALORIES
LUNCH	
DINNER	
(SNACK)	
	TOTAL

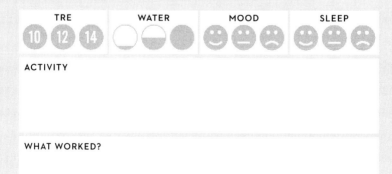

TRE   10   12   14

WATER

MOOD

SLEEP

ACTIVITY

WHAT WORKED?

Week Nine
THURSDAY

BREAKFAST	CALORIES
LUNCH	
DINNER	
(SNACK)	
	TOTAL

TRE	WATER	MOOD	SLEEP
10 12 14			

ACTIVITY

WHAT WORKED?

Prioritise sleep.

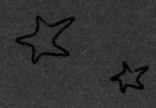

Most people need at least
seven to eight hours' sleep
a night and if you get by
on less than that you are
more likely to experience
hunger and cravings,
particularly for high-carb,
high-calorie foods.

Week Nine
FRIDAY

NON-FASTING DAY   800 DAY

BREAKFAST	CALORIES

LUNCH	

DINNER	

(SNACK)	

	TOTAL

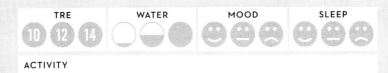

TRE	WATER	MOOD	SLEEP
10 12 14			

ACTIVITY

WHAT WORKED?

155

Week Nine
SATURDAY

○ NON-FASTING DAY   ○ 800 DAY

BREAKFAST	CALORIES

LUNCH	

DINNER	

(SNACK)	

	TOTAL

TRE	WATER	MOOD	SLEEP
10 12 14	◐	😊 😐 ☹️	😊 😐 ☹️

ACTIVITY

WHAT WORKED?

156

Week Nine
SUNDAY

BREAKFAST	CALORIES

LUNCH	

DINNER	

(SNACK)	

TOTAL

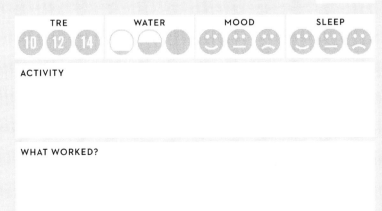

TRE

WATER

MOOD

SLEEP

ACTIVITY

WHAT WORKED?

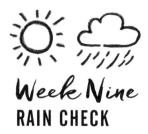

Week Nine
RAIN CHECK

Not long to go! Losing weight will mean that you sleep better, which means you will be less likely to feel those sleep-deprived bingeing urges. Intermittent fasting has been shown to improve mood, probably by boosting levels of the hormone BDNF, which helps protect and build brain and nerve cells.

Your microbiome (those trillions of bugs in your gut) are also likely to be in better shape with your healthier Med-style diet. This is well known to lead to improvement in mood, reduction in anxiety and better sleep.

If, however, stress and poor sleep are still an issue, it might be helpful to look at practical ways of managing these or getting extra support to do so. Being tired and anxious can sabotage all the best plans.

"I've never felt better in my life. I refuse to be a slave to my health issues. I took my life back with this programme. Thank you Dr Mosley and team for this life-changing experience. I'm a Mediterranean Diet girl for life!" Ginger

WEIGHT	NUMBER OF 800 DAYS THIS WEEK
WAIST	NUMBER OF NON-FASTING DAYS THIS WEEK

FOOD: WHAT WORKED AND WHAT DO YOU PLAN TO CHANGE?

ACTIVITY: WHAT WORKED AND WHAT DO YOU PLAN TO CHANGE?

WATER INTAKE	OVERALL MOOD	OVERALL SLEEP

HOW ARE YOU COPING AND WHAT DO YOU PLAN TO CHANGE?

WHAT ARE YOU MOST PROUD OF?

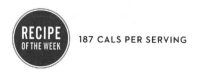 187 CALS PER SERVING

Roasted vegetable soup

Fabulously filling, the flavour is intensified by roasting the veg.

SERVES 4

1 medium celeriac (around 650g),
    peeled and cut into roughly 3cm chunks
2 medium carrots (around 200g),
    trimmed and cut into roughly 3cm chunks
1 large red pepper, deseeded and cut into roughly 4cm chunks
1 medium onion, peeled and cut into 12 wedges
2 tbsp olive oil
500ml vegetable or chicken stock (made with 1 stock cube)
25g flaked almonds, ideally toasted, to serve

1. Preheat the oven to 200°C/fan 180°C/Gas 4.

2. Place the vegetables in a large bowl and toss with the oil.
Scatter over a large baking tray and cook in the oven for about
35 minutes, turning all the veg after 15 minutes, or until softened
and lightly browned without being crisp.

3. Transfer the vegetables to a large saucepan and add the stock.
Blitz with a stick blender until smooth.

4. Add a further 600ml cold water and bring to a gentle simmer,
stirring regularly. Add a little extra water, if needed, to reach
your preferred consistency. Season to taste with salt and pepper.

5. Ladle the soup into warmed bowls and top with toasted
flaked almonds to serve.

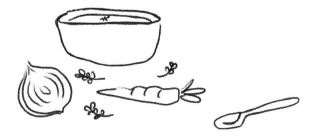

Week Ten
TARGETS & AIMS

WRITE DOWN YOUR WEIGHT

ANY BIG EVENTS OR OCCASIONS YOU NEED TO FACTOR IN?

WHAT ARE YOUR GOALS THIS WEEK?

WHICH WILL BE YOUR FASTING DAYS?

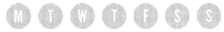

Be kind to yourself. Sometimes you will give in to temptations – it's only human.

FOOD PLANNER

Plan your meals for the week ahead

	MONDAY	TUESDAY	WEDNESDAY	THURSDAY
BREAKFAST				
LUNCH				
DINNER				
(SNACK)				
CALORIES				

FRIDAY	SATURDAY	SUNDAY	
			TOTAL CALORIES

SHOPPING LIST

NOTES

Week Ten
MONDAY

NON-FASTING DAY ◯   800 DAY ◯

BREAKFAST	CALORIES
LUNCH	
DINNER	
(SNACK)	
	TOTAL

TRE	WATER	MOOD	SLEEP
	◯ ◑ ●		

ACTIVITY

WHAT WORKED?

Week Ten
TUESDAY

NON-FASTING DAY   800 DAY

BREAKFAST	CALORIES

LUNCH	

DINNER	

(SNACK)	

TOTAL

TRE	WATER	MOOD	SLEEP
10 12 14	◯ ◒ ●	☺ 😐 ☹	☺ 😐 ☹

ACTIVITY

WHAT WORKED?

167

Week Ten
WEDNESDAY

BREAKFAST	CALORIES
LUNCH	
DINNER	
(SNACK)	
	TOTAL

TRE	WATER	MOOD	SLEEP
10 12 14			

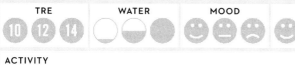

ACTIVITY

WHAT WORKED?

Week Ten
THURSDAY

BREAKFAST	CALORIES

LUNCH	

DINNER	

(SNACK)	

TOTAL

TRE	WATER	MOOD	SLEEP
10 12 14			

ACTIVITY

WHAT WORKED?

Try this simple breathing exercise.

Find a quiet room and sit with your eyes closed. Breathe in to a count of four through your nose and then, without pausing or holding your breath, let the air flow gently out, counting from one to four. Keep doing this for 3 to 5 minutes.

Week Ten
FRIDAY

NON-FASTING DAY   800 DAY

	CALORIES
BREAKFAST	
LUNCH	
DINNER	
(SNACK)	

TOTAL

TRE	WATER	MOOD	SLEEP

ACTIVITY

WHAT WORKED?

Week Ten
SATURDAY

NON-FASTING DAY   800 DAY

BREAKFAST	CALORIES

LUNCH	

DINNER	

(SNACK)	

TOTAL

TRE	WATER	MOOD	SLEEP
10 12 14			

ACTIVITY

WHAT WORKED?

Week Ten
SUNDAY

NON-FASTING DAY   800 DAY

BREAKFAST	CALORIES

LUNCH	

DINNER	

(SNACK)	

TOTAL

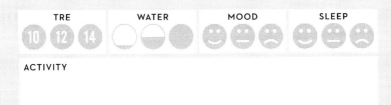

TRE	WATER	MOOD	SLEEP
10 12 14	○ ◐ ●	🙂 😐 ☹️	🙂 😐 ☹️

ACTIVITY

WHAT WORKED?

173

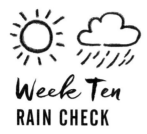

Week Ten
RAIN CHECK

At this stage in the programme, you will feel like an old hand. Not only will you be cooking and eating differently, but all sorts of other lifestyle habits will have changed, too. Keep up the good work. Get outside as much as you can. Treat yourself to new clothes. Revisit your goals and celebrate your achievements!

"You can use the recipes for the whole family so it doesn't have to be too much work." Dale

WEIGHT	NUMBER OF 800 DAYS THIS WEEK
WAIST	NUMBER OF NON-FASTING DAYS THIS WEEK

FOOD: WHAT WORKED AND WHAT DO YOU PLAN TO CHANGE?

ACTIVITY: WHAT WORKED AND WHAT DO YOU PLAN TO CHANGE?

WATER INTAKE	OVERALL MOOD	OVERALL SLEEP
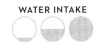	😊 😐 ☹️	😊 😐 ☹️

HOW ARE YOU COPING AND WHAT DO YOU PLAN TO CHANGE?

WHAT ARE YOU MOST PROUD OF?

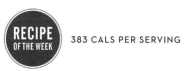 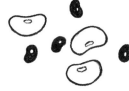

RECIPE OF THE WEEK 383 CALS PER SERVING

Slow-cooked spicy pork & beans

High in flavour, low in sugar, this will fill you up and keep your gut healthy, too. Serve with freshly cooked green vegetables or a large mixed salad. This is also good served with cauli-rice (see page 80).

SERVES 3
2 tbsp olive oil
1 medium onion, peeled and thinly sliced
2 pork shoulder steaks (around 375g),
    trimmed and cut into roughly 3cm chunks
1 tsp hot smoked paprika
½ tsp ground cumin
½ tsp ground coriander
1 × 400g can chopped tomatoes
1 × 400g can black beans, or red kidney beans,
    drained and rinsed
1 chicken or pork stock cube
125g full-fat live Greek yoghurt, to serve

1. Preheat the oven to 170°C/fan 150°C/Gas 3.

2. Heat the oil in a flame-proof casserole, then add the onion and pork, season with ground black pepper and fry over a medium heat for 5 minutes, or until lightly browned, stirring occasionally.

3. Add the spices and cook for a few seconds more, stirring. Tip the tomatoes and beans into the pan. Refill the tomato can with water and pour into the pan as well. Add the crumbled stock cube and stir well. Bring to a simmer.

4. Cover with a lid and cook in the oven for 1½–2 hours, or until the pork is tender and the sauce is thick. Serve topped with yoghurt.

COOK'S TIP: Any leftover portions are great reheated and served in lettuce wraps, or freeze for up to 3 months.

NON-FAST DAY: Increase the portion size and serve on a slice of seeded brown sourdough bread.

Week Eleven
TARGETS & AIMS

WRITE DOWN YOUR WEIGHT

ANY BIG EVENTS OR OCCASIONS YOU NEED TO FACTOR IN?

WHAT ARE YOUR GOALS THIS WEEK?

WHICH WILL BE YOUR FASTING DAYS?

A year from now you will wish you had started today.
Karen Lamb

FOOD PLANNER

Plan your meals for the week ahead

	MONDAY	TUESDAY	WEDNESDAY	THURSDAY
BREAKFAST				
LUNCH				
DINNER				
(SNACK)				
CALORIES				

FRIDAY	SATURDAY	SUNDAY	
			TOTAL CALORIES

SHOPPING LIST

NOTES

Week Eleven
MONDAY

○ NON-FASTING DAY   ○ 800 DAY

BREAKFAST	CALORIES
LUNCH	
DINNER	
(SNACK)	
	TOTAL

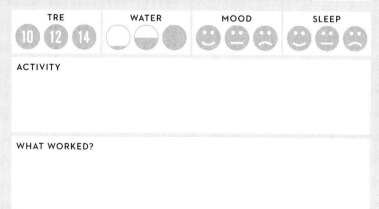

TRE	WATER	MOOD	SLEEP
10 12 14	○ ◑ ●	☺ ☺ ☹	☺ ☺ ☹

ACTIVITY

WHAT WORKED?

Week Eleven
TUESDAY

BREAKFAST	CALORIES
LUNCH	
DINNER	
(SNACK)	
	TOTAL

TRE 10 12 14

WATER

MOOD

SLEEP

ACTIVITY

WHAT WORKED?

Week Eleven
WEDNESDAY

NON-FASTING DAY ○ 800 DAY ○

BREAKFAST	CALORIES
LUNCH	
DINNER	
(SNACK)	
	TOTAL

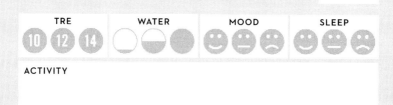

TRE 10 12 14

WATER

MOOD

SLEEP

ACTIVITY

WHAT WORKED?

Week Eleven
THURSDAY

NON-FASTING DAY   800 DAY

BREAKFAST	CALORIES
LUNCH	
DINNER	
(SNACK)	

TOTAL

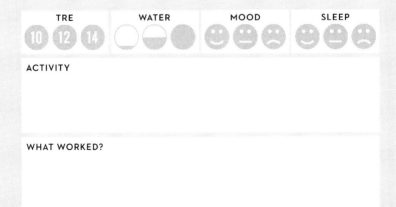

TRE   10 12 14

WATER

MOOD

SLEEP

ACTIVITY

WHAT WORKED?

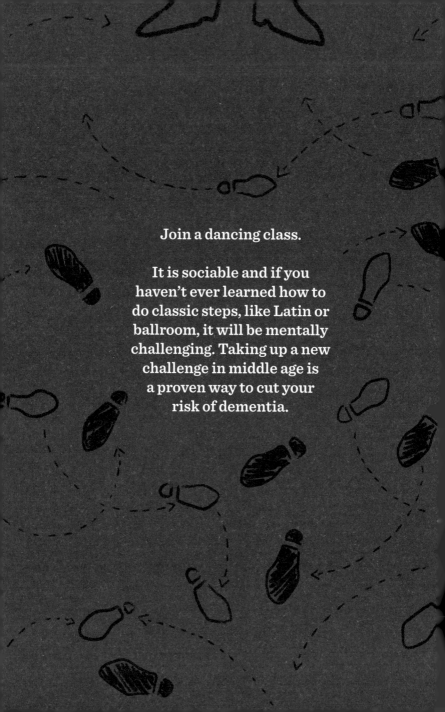

Join a dancing class.

It is sociable and if you haven't ever learned how to do classic steps, like Latin or ballroom, it will be mentally challenging. Taking up a new challenge in middle age is a proven way to cut your risk of dementia.

Week Eleven
FRIDAY

○ NON-FASTING DAY   ○ 800 DAY

	CALORIES
BREAKFAST	
LUNCH	
DINNER	
(SNACK)	
TOTAL	

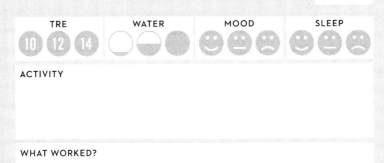

TRE   10   12   14

WATER

MOOD

SLEEP

ACTIVITY

WHAT WORKED?

Week Eleven
SATURDAY

NON-FASTING DAY   800 DAY

BREAKFAST	CALORIES

LUNCH	

DINNER	

(SNACK)	

TOTAL

TRE   10   12   14   WATER   MOOD   SLEEP

ACTIVITY

WHAT WORKED?

Week Eleven
SUNDAY

NON-FASTING DAY   800 DAY

BREAKFAST	CALORIES

LUNCH	

DINNER	

(SNACK)	

TOTAL

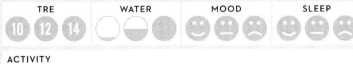

TRE   WATER   MOOD   SLEEP

ACTIVITY

WHAT WORKED?

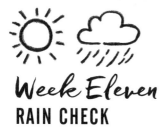

Week Eleven
RAIN CHECK

You are so nearly there now. Having lost weight, you will not only feel better and have more energy, you will also have gained future health benefits, which should be very motivating. By losing visceral fat (the hidden interior fat) and changing what you eat, you will have reduced your risk of many chronic diseases. People with high blood pressure should be seeing significant improvements and may have cut their medication.

Those with type 2 diabetes or pre-diabetes may have seen their blood sugar levels returned to normal, without medication. You have embraced a new way of life. For many people, simply sticking to a relatively low-carb Med-style diet and managing portion control is enough.

"I cannot tell you how happy I am, I've been type 2 diabetic for 5 years and they were about to start me on medication. I honestly feel like I've been saved from a lifetime of ill health – this diet has been the best life change I have ever made and Dr Michael Mosley deserves a knighthood for it." Debby

WEIGHT	NUMBER OF 800 DAYS THIS WEEK
WAIST	NUMBER OF NON-FASTING DAYS THIS WEEK

FOOD: WHAT WORKED AND WHAT DO YOU PLAN TO CHANGE?

ACTIVITY: WHAT WORKED AND WHAT DO YOU PLAN TO CHANGE?

WATER INTAKE	OVERALL MOOD	OVERALL SLEEP
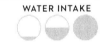		

HOW ARE YOU COPING AND WHAT DO YOU PLAN TO CHANGE?

WHAT ARE YOU MOST PROUD OF?

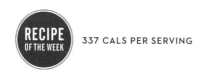

Fluffy smoked salmon omelette with spinach

We love this light and fluffy omelette – easy, tasty and super healthy. Ideal for breakfast or enjoy it as a light meal with a colourful salad or with half a plate of non-starchy vegetables, such as broccoli.

SERVES 1
2 large eggs
1 heaped tsp butter or 1 tsp olive oil
50g smoked salmon (around 2 slices), cut into strips
large handful young spinach leaves (around 50g)

1. Break the eggs into a small bowl, add some freshly ground black pepper and whisk well.

2. Melt the butter or heat the oil in a medium non-stick frying pan over a medium heat.

3. Add the salmon and spinach and cook together for about 1½ minutes, or until the salmon is pale pink and the spinach softened, stirring regularly.

4. Tip the eggs into the pan and allow to spread over the salmon and spinach. Cook for a few seconds, then begin to bring the sides of the egg in towards the centre of the pan, allowing the uncooked egg to run back out. Work your way around the pan, heaping the softly cooked egg up in the centre. After about 1 minute, when the egg is just cooked, slide on to a warmed plate and serve.

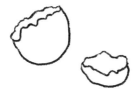

Week Twelve
TARGETS & AIMS

WRITE DOWN YOUR WEIGHT

ANY BIG EVENTS OR OCCASIONS YOU NEED TO FACTOR IN?

WHAT ARE YOUR GOALS THIS WEEK?

WHICH WILL BE YOUR FASTING DAYS?

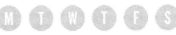

There is only one time that is important – Now! It is the most important time because it is the only time when we have any power. *Leo Tolstoy*

FOOD PLANNER

Plan your meals for the week ahead

	MONDAY	TUESDAY	WEDNESDAY	THURSDAY
BREAKFAST				
LUNCH				
DINNER				
(SNACK)				
CALORIES				

FRIDAY	SATURDAY	SUNDAY	
			TOTAL CALORIES

SHOPPING LIST

NOTES

Week Twelve
MONDAY

BREAKFAST	CALORIES

LUNCH	

DINNER	

(SNACK)	

TOTAL

TRE	WATER	MOOD	SLEEP
10 12 14	◯ ◖ ●	☺ 😐 ☹	☺ 😐 ☹

ACTIVITY

WHAT WORKED?

Week Twelve
TUESDAY

NON-FASTING DAY   800 DAY

	CALORIES
BREAKFAST	
LUNCH	
DINNER	
(SNACK)	
TOTAL	

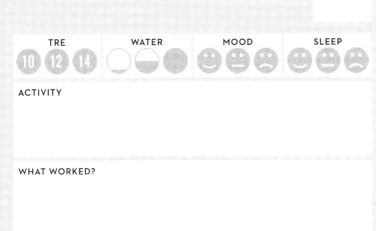

TRE   10   12   14

WATER

MOOD

SLEEP

ACTIVITY

WHAT WORKED?

Week Twelve
WEDNESDAY

NON-FASTING DAY   800 DAY

BREAKFAST	CALORIES
LUNCH	
DINNER	
(SNACK)	
	TOTAL

TRE	WATER	MOOD	SLEEP
10 12 14			

ACTIVITY

WHAT WORKED?

Week Twelve
THURSDAY

NON-FASTING DAY   800 DAY

BREAKFAST	CALORIES

LUNCH	

DINNER	

(SNACK)

TOTAL

TRE   WATER   MOOD   SLEEP
10 12 14

ACTIVITY

WHAT WORKED?

Remind yourself why
you are doing this.

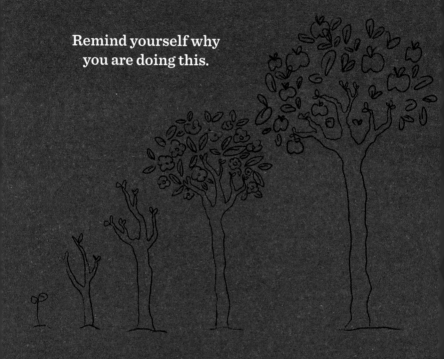

"I want to live to a healthy old age,
enjoying life with friends and family."
Whatever your motives, remind
yourself of them from time to time.
And remember that, as with adopting
any new habit, it really does get
easier with time.

Week Twelve
FRIDAY

BREAKFAST	CALORIES

LUNCH	

DINNER	

(SNACK)	

TOTAL

TRE   10 12 14

WATER

MOOD

SLEEP

ACTIVITY

WHAT WORKED?

Week Twelve
SATURDAY

○ NON-FASTING DAY   ○ 800 DAY

BREAKFAST	CALORIES

LUNCH	

DINNER	

(SNACK)	

	TOTAL

TRE	WATER	MOOD	SLEEP
10 12 14	○ ◑ ●	☺ 😐 ☹	☺ 😐 ☹

ACTIVITY

WHAT WORKED?

204

Week Twelve
SUNDAY

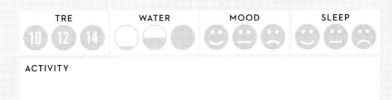

NON-FASTING DAY   800 DAY

BREAKFAST	CALORIES

LUNCH	

DINNER	

(SNACK)	

TOTAL

TRE   WATER   MOOD   SLEEP

ACTIVITY

WHAT WORKED?

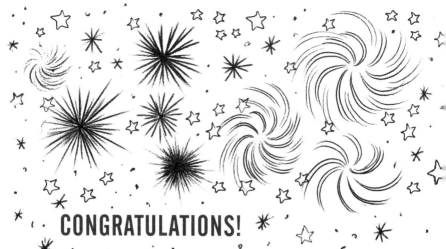

CONGRATULATIONS!

Well done for making it through the 12 weeks. We hope you have achieved some or even all of your aims on the Fast 800 and that the journal has helped to keep you on track.

You will have made significant changes by now, and should feel happier, brighter and lighter – more confident and back in control. Many of you will be ready to settle in to the low-carb Med-style Way of Life. However, if you have further to go, you may want to stick to the New 5:2 approach until you reach your goal. You can download supplementary daily journal pages from www.thefast800.com, where you will find lots of extra recipes, further reading and resources, including an online programme offering you more support.

Before continuing with the fasting programme, we would also suggest you consult a doctor or other health professional.

You may worry about occasional lapses – these are inevitable so don't beat yourself up. But if you return to your old ways, you will probably return to your pre-diet body. Do your best to avoid temptation – check that junk food, and watch out for portion creep and snacking! And if things slip, you know what to do – just go back on to the Fast 800! A 2kg weight increase should trigger your attention. You can do it and it's best to get back on track early if you can.

Twelve weeks on! How have you got on?

WHAT DIFFERENCE HAS THE FAST 800 MADE TO YOU?

HOW CLOSE HAVE YOU GOT TO YOUR GOALS?

HOW ARE YOU GOING TO CELEBRATE AND SHARE YOUR SUCCESS?

IF YOU HAVEN'T REACHED YOUR GOALS, WHAT DO YOU PLAN
TO DO MOVING FORWARDS?

HOW ARE YOU GOING TO MAINTAIN YOUR NEW HEALTHY STATE?

Record your latest statistics and feel proud! Check
back to goal setting (page 15) to see how far you've come.
Continue to weigh yourself weekly as it's much easier
to keep on track if you catch the weight gain early!

	CURRENT	ORIGINAL
WEIGHT		
BMI		
WAIST		
HbA1C		
OTHER		

"The best surprise was that my husband also loved the food. He even took to cooking some of the meals. Big bonus!" Karen

"This recipe book is the 'Holy Grail' we've been looking for." B.

"You have literally saved my life. It took 3 months and I'm cured and I am spreading the word. I just wanted to say thank you." Dave

"It's evidence based and very informative. With all the conflicting advice out there about diet and lifestyle it was great to follow a plan backed up by the latest research. It's a wonderful lifestyle overhaul not just a 'diet'." Caroline

"You don't need a gym membership. I did my workout in the kitchen!" Jane

"I've lost 2 and half stone in 3 months following this diet, which for a woman in her late forties with an 8-hour-a-day desk job, I think is impressive! I feel so much happier and healthier." Julie

"I lost 5kg and I feel so much healthier. I've learnt so much; a wonderful lifestyle overhaul." Caroline

"Wow. I loved the impact this plan had on my insulin. Finally, a plan that works." Nina

"The fasting blood test I had after 5 weeks proved just how healthy it is, I've never had such good results. That blood test is what is spurring me on. I am so glad I took the plunge." Valerie

"Five months after starting The Fast 800 I reached my target of 3 stones lost. I've gone on to lose a few more pounds to bring my total to 45lbs. I have a whole new figure, necessitating a whole new wardrobe! I feel wonderful, am much more active, and have no joint pain. This WORKS!" Yvonne

"I have just finished my 8 weeks and have lost 23lbs, which 2 months ago I didn't think was achievable." Kate

"I was so surprised by how good the recipes were – couldn't believe I was on a health plan!" Dale

"I totally recommend the online plan and the recipe book and will continue to use the recipes because they are just so good." Dory

BONUS RECIPES

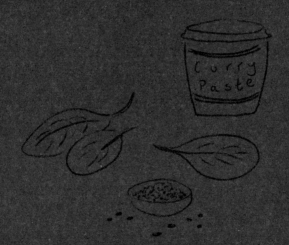

Curry Three Ways

The three quick and easy curries overleaf are all based on the delicious, richly flavoured curry base below, suggested by my colleague Parmi. Her mother would cook this paste daily but, as a working mother, Parmi prefers to cook it in batches. It's far tastier than shop-bought curry pastes and lower in sugar, too.

BASIC CURRY PASTE. MAKES 3 BATCHES
4 tbsp coconut, rapeseed or olive oil
3 medium onions, peeled and finely chopped
5 tsp curry powder (hot, medium or mild, to taste)
25g fresh root ginger, peeled and finely chopped
3 large garlic cloves (about 10g), peeled and finely chopped
20g fresh coriander, roughly chopped

1. Heat the oil in a large non-stick saucepan over a low-medium heat. Add the onions, cover with a lid and cook gently for 15–20 minutes, stirring occasionally.

2. Add the curry powder and continue to cook for a few seconds. Stir in the ginger and garlic and cook for a further 8–10 minutes, stirring regularly. Add 1 tablespoon water halfway through the cooking time, and again if the spices begin to stick.

3. Stir in the coriander and a further 3–4 tablespoons water to loosen and cook for 1–2 minutes, or until softened, stirring constantly. Remove the pan from the heat.

4. Use a stick blender, or cool for a few minutes and transfer to a food processor, and blitz into a paste. Season well with salt and ground black pepper.

5. Divide into 3 batches (each will serve 2 people) and use immediately, or cool and store in the fridge or freezer.

Red lentil dhal

SERVES 2
80g dried red split lentils
1 batch basic curry paste (page 211)
1 tbsp coconut, rapeseed or olive oil
1 small onion, peeled and sliced into rings
fresh coriander leaves, to serve (optional)

1. Place the lentils, curry paste and 400ml water in a medium non-stick saucepan. Bring to a simmer and cook for 15–20 minutes, or until the lentils are very soft, stirring occasionally. Add a splash more water, if needed. The dhal should be very soft and not too thick.

2. Meanwhile, heat the oil in a small frying pan and gently fry the onion until pale golden, turning frequently. Set aside.

3. When you are ready to serve, spoon the onion rings on top of the dhal and scatter with coriander leaves, if using.

325 CALS PER SERVING

Spinach & paneer curry

SERVES 2
1 batch basic curry paste (page 211)
1 × 400g can chopped tomatoes
2 generous handfuls young spinach leaves (around 75g)
100g paneer cheese, cut into roughly 1.5cm cubes

1. Place the curry paste and tomatoes in a large non-stick frying pan and bring to a gentle simmer over a medium heat. Cook for 5 minutes, stirring regularly.

2. Stir in 200ml water, then the spinach, a handful at a time, and simmer gently for 2–3 minutes, stirring.

3. Add the cheese and cook for 2–3 minutes more, or until hot.

Chicken & chickpea curry

SERVES 3
1 tbsp coconut, rapeseed or olive oil
4 boneless, skinless chicken thighs (about 450g),
    trimmed and quartered
1 batch basic curry paste (page 211)
1 × 400g can chopped tomatoes
1 × 210g can chickpeas in water

1. Heat the oil in a large non-stick saucepan over a medium heat. Add the chicken and fry for 5 minutes, or until lightly coloured, turning occasionally.

2. Stir in the curry paste and cook for 2–3 minutes more, stirring regularly.

3. Add the tomatoes, half fill the can with water and pour this into the pan as well. Add the chickpeas without draining them and bring to a gentle simmer.

4. Cover loosely with a lid and cook for about 30 minutes, stirring occasionally, until the chicken is tender and the sauce has thickened. Add a little extra water if needed and season well with salt and pepper.

COOK'S TIP: Serve with cauli-rice (see page 80).

NON-FAST DAY: Serve with a drizzle of full-fat live Greek yoghurt or raitha and include 2–3 tablespoons brown or wild rice.

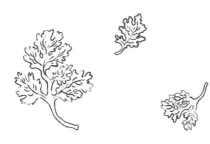

Winter slaw

A colourful and versatile crunchy slaw. It lasts well in the
fridge for 2–3 days.

SERVES 4
¼ medium red cabbage (around 225g),
    cored and shredded as finely as possible
½ medium celeriac (around 300g), peeled and
    coarsely grated (around 225g prepped weight)
1 medium carrot (around 115g),
    trimmed and coarsely grated
3 spring onions, trimmed and finely sliced
50g mixed nuts, roughly chopped
20g mixed seeds (around 2 tbsp)

For the dressing
150g full-fat live Greek yoghurt
50g good-quality mayonnaise (not low-fat)
2 tsp Dijon mustard

1. To make the dressing, mix the yoghurt, mayonnaise,
mustard and 4 tablespoons cold water in a large bowl.

2. Add all the vegetables to the dressing and toss together well.
Sprinkle with the nuts and seeds, season with salt and plenty
of freshly ground black pepper. Toss again to serve on its own
or with one of the following serving suggestions:

50g (roughly 2 slices) ham per person for an additional 54 calories

50g (roughly 2 slices) cooked roast beef per person for an
additional 100 calories

1 smoked mackerel fillet (around 70g skin on) per person for an
additional 221 calories

60g sliced halloumi cheese, griddled or fried in a dry pan, per person
for an additional 237 calories

1 large hard-boiled egg per person, for an additional 92 calories

Very low-calorie instant miso soup

When Michael did a very low-calorie, four-day fast to reverse his diabetes, this was his saviour. Perfect low-cal comfort food and surprisingly filling.

SERVES 1
1 tbsp miso (from a jar)
2 spring onions, trimmed and finely sliced
1 tsp finely grated fresh root ginger
½ garlic clove, peeled and very finely sliced
good pinch crushed dried chilli flakes,
**   or ½ small red chilli, finely sliced**
2 handfuls young spinach leaves, tender kale leaves,
**   shredded watercress or finely sliced pak choi**
dark soy sauce, to taste

1. Put the miso in a medium saucepan and add 500ml (around 2 mugfuls) just-boiled water.

2. Stir in the spring onions, ginger, garlic and chilli and bring to a gentle simmer. Stir in the leaves and cook for 1–2 minutes more, or until softened.

3. Serve in a deep bowl, seasoned with soy sauce, to taste.

COOK'S TIP: Add 3–4 very thinly sliced mushrooms to the pan, if you like – mushrooms add extra fibre and nutrients with minimal added calories.

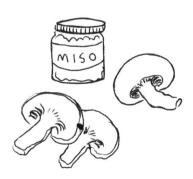

NOTES

NOTES

NOTES

NOTES

DR MICHAEL MOSLEY is a science presenter, journalist and executive producer. After training to be a doctor at the Royal Free Hospital in London, he spent 25 years at the BBC, where he made numerous science documentaries. Now freelance, he is the author of several bestselling books, *The Fast Diet*, *The 8-Week Blood Sugar Diet* and *The Clever Guts Diet*. He is married with four children.

DR CLARE BAILEY, wife of Michael Mosley, is a GP who has supported hundreds of patients to lose weight, reduce their blood sugars and put their diabetes into remission at her surgery in Buckinghamshire. She is the author of the bestselling *8-Week Blood Sugar Diet Recipe Book*, *Clever Guts Diet Recipe Book* and *The Fast 800 Recipe Book*. @drclarebailey

JUSTINE PATTISON is one of the UK's leading healthy-eating recipe writers. She has published numerous books, makes regular appearances on television, can often be heard on the radio and contributes to many top magazines, newspapers and websites. www.justinepattison.com

Published in 2019 by
Short Books, Unit 316,
ScreenWorks,
22 Highbury Grove,
London, N5 2ER

10 9 8 7 6 5 4 3 2 1

A CIP catalogue record for this book is available from the British Library.

ISBN: 978-1-78072-416-4

Design by Smith & Gilmour
Illustrations by Emily Mosley
Recipe consultancy by Justine Pattison

Printed and bound by CPI Group (UK) Ltd, Croydon, CR0 4YY

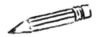